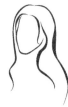

## This Book Belongs to:

_____

📞 _____

✉ _____

_____

## Emergency Contacts

_____

_____

_____

_____

_____

_____

_____

# Treatment History

DATE: ☐ Medication
☐ Non Medication

Description:

_____

Result:

_____

DATE: ☐ Medication
☐ Non Medication

Description:

_____

Result:

_____

DATE: ☐ Medication
☐ Non Medication

Description:

_____

Result:

_____

DATE: ☐ Medication
☐ Non Medication

Description:

_____

Result:

_____

DATE: ☐ Medication
☐ Non Medication

Description:

_____

Result:

_____

# Treatment History

DATE:      ☐ Medication
             ☐ Non Medication

Description:

Result:

DATE:      ☐ Medication
             ☐ Non Medication

Description:

Result:

DATE:      ☐ Medication
             ☐ Non Medication

Description:

Result:

DATE:      ☐ Medication
             ☐ Non Medication

Description:

Result:

DATE:      ☐ Medication
             ☐ Non Medication

Description:

Result:

# Treatment History

DATE:    ☐ Medication
           ☐ Non Medication

Description:

Result:

DATE:    ☐ Medication
           ☐ Non Medication

Description:

Result:

DATE:    ☐ Medication
           ☐ Non Medication

Description:

Result:

DATE:    ☐ Medication
           ☐ Non Medication

Description:

Result:

DATE:    ☐ Medication
           ☐ Non Medication

Description:

Result:

# Location of headache

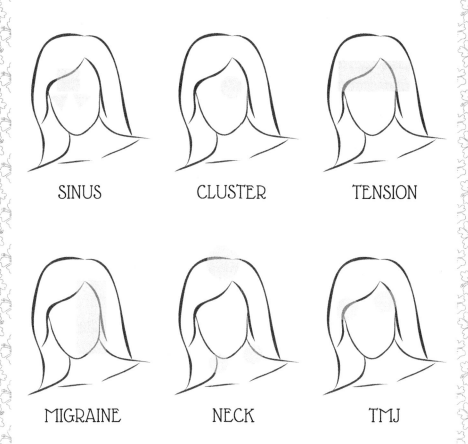

SINUS

CLUSTER

TENSION

MIGRAINE

NECK

TMJ

"Some pain you can distance yourself from, but a headache sits right where you live." ~ Mark Lawrence

Date:      Start Time:      Severity/Intensity

End Time:    ⓪ ① ② ③ ④ ⑤

## Location of headache

○ SINUS   ○ CLUSTER   ○ TENSION    ○ MIGRAINE   ○ NECK   ○ TMJ

## Other Symptoms _____

_____

| Triggers | | Weather | Mood before |
|---|---|---|---|

### Triggers
- ○ Alcohol
- ○ Caffeine
- ○ Hunger
- ○ Tiredness
- ○ Allergies
- ○ Chocolate
- ○ Other: _____

- ○ Stress at Home
- ○ Stress at Work
- ○ Eyestrain
- ○ Weather
- ○ PMS
- ○ Odor

### Weather
- ☐ SUNNY
- ☐ CLOUDY
- ☐ RAINY

Temp: _____

### Mood before Headache:
- ○ Happy
- ○ Normal
- ○ Indifferent
- ○ Nervous
- ○ Tired
- ○ Sad

Other: _____

## Medications & Supplements

_____

_____

_____

_____

_____

### Other Relief Methods:
- ☐ ICE    ☐ RELAX
- ☐ HEAT   ☐ OTHER
- ☐ BED REST
- ☐ MASSAGE
- ☐ LOWER LIGHTS

## Food Intake _____

_____

_____

_____

_____

_____

## Hours of Sleep

## Water Intake

🍶 🍶 🍶 🍶 🍶

🍶 🍶 🍶 🍶 🍶

**Date:**     **Start Time:**     **Severity/Intensity**

**End Time:**     (0) (1) (2) (3) (4) (5)

## Location of headache
○ SINUS   ○ CLUSTER   ○ TENSION   ○ MIGRAINE   ○ NECK   ○ TMJ

## Other Symptoms _____

_____

### Triggers
○ Alcohol     ○ Stress at Home
○ Caffeine    ○ Stress at Work
○ Hunger      ○ Eyestrain
○ Tiredness   ○ Weather
○ Allergies   ○ PMS
○ Chocolate   ○ Odor
○ Other: _____

### ☁ Weather
☐ SUNNY
☐ CLOUDY
☐ RAINY
Temp: _____

### Mood before Headache:
○ Happy
○ Normal
○ Indifferent
○ Nervous
○ Tired
○ Sad
Other:
_____

## 💊 Medications & Supplements
_____
_____
_____
_____
_____

### Other Relief Methods:
☐ ICE      ☐ RELAX
☐ HEAT     ☐ OTHER
☐ BED REST
☐ MASSAGE
☐ LOWER LIGHTS

## 🍳 Food Intake _____
_____
_____
_____
_____
_____

### ☾ Hours of Sleep
_____

### ○ Water Intake
🍶 🍶 🍶 🍶 🍶

🍶 🍶 🍶 🍶 🍶

# Notes

_____

_____

_____

_____

_____

_____

_____

_____

_____

_____

_____

_____

_____

_____

_____

_____

_____

_____

Date:     Start Time:     Severity/Intensity

End Time:     (0) (1) (2) (3) (4) (5)

## Location of headache

○ SINUS ○ CLUSTER ○ TENSION ○ MIGRAINE ○ NECK ○ TMJ

## Other Symptoms _____

_____

### Triggers

○ Alcohol ○ Stress at Home
○ Caffeine ○ Stress at Work
○ Hunger ○ Eyestrain
○ Tiredness ○ Weather
○ Allergies ○ PMS
○ Chocolate ○ Odor
○ Other: _____

### Weather

☐ SUNNY
☐ CLOUDY
☐ RAINY

Temp: _____

### Mood before Headache:

○ Happy
○ Normal
○ Indifferent
○ Nervous
○ Tired
○ Sad

Other: _____

## Medications & Supplements

_____
_____
_____
_____
_____

## Other Relief Methods:

☐ ICE    ☐ RELAX
☐ HEAT ☐ OTHER
☐ BED REST
☐ MASSAGE
☐ LOWER LIGHTS

## Food Intake _____

_____
_____
_____
_____
_____
_____

## Hours of Sleep

_____

## Water Intake

Date:      Start Time:      Severity/Intensity

End Time:    ⓪ ① ② ③ ④ ⑤

## Location of headache
○ SINUS   ○ CLUSTER   ○ TENSION   ○ MIGRAINE   ○ NECK   ○ TMJ

## Other Symptoms _____

_____

| Triggers | | Weather | Mood before |
|---|---|---|---|

### Triggers
○ Alcohol    ○ Stress at Home
○ Caffeine    ○ Stress at Work
○ Hunger    ○ Eyestrain
○ Tiredness    ○ Weather
○ Allergies    ○ PMS
○ Chocolate    ○ Odor
○ Other: _____

### Weather
☐ SUNNY
☐ CLOUDY
☐ RAINY
Temp: _____

### Mood before Headache:
○ Happy
○ Normal
○ Indifferent
○ Nervous
○ Tired
○ Sad
Other:
_____

## Medications & Supplements

_____
_____
_____
_____
_____

### Other Relief Methods:
☐ ICE    ☐ RELAX
☐ HEAT    ☐ OTHER
☐ BED REST
☐ MASSAGE
☐ LOWER LIGHTS

## Food Intake _____

_____
_____
_____
_____
_____

## Hours of Sleep

_____

## Water Intake

# Notes

Date:      Start Time:      Severity/Intensity

End Time:    ⓪ ① ② ③ ④ ⑤

## Location of headache

○ SINUS ○ CLUSTER ○ TENSION ○ MIGRAINE ○ NECK ○ TMJ

## Other Symptoms _____

_____

### Triggers

○ Alcohol ○ Stress at Home
○ Caffeine ○ Stress at Work
○ Hunger ○ Eyestrain
○ Tiredness ○ Weather
○ Allergies ○ PMS
○ Chocolate ○ Odor
○ Other: _____

### ☁Weather

☐ SUNNY
☐ CLOUDY
☐ RAINY

Temp: _____

### Mood before Headache:

○ Happy
○ Normal
○ Indifferent
○ Nervous
○ Tired
○ Sad

Other: _____

## Medications & Supplements

_____
_____
_____
_____
_____

## Other Relief Methods:

☐ ICE ☐ RELAX
☐ HEAT ☐ OTHER
☐ BED REST
☐ MASSAGE
☐ LOWER LIGHTS

## Food Intake _____

_____
_____
_____
_____
_____
_____

## ☾ Hours of Sleep

_____

## ◊ Water Intake

## Notes

Date:　　　Start Time:　　　Severity/Intensity

End Time:　　　(0) (1) (2) (3) (4) (5)

## Location of headache

○ SINUS ○ CLUSTER ○ TENSION ○ MIGRAINE ○ NECK ○ TMJ

## Other Symptoms _____

_____

### Triggers

○ Alcohol ○ Stress at Home
○ Caffeine ○ Stress at Work
○ Hunger ○ Eyestrain
○ Tiredness ○ Weather
○ Allergies ○ PMS
○ Chocolate ○ Odor
○ Other: _____

### Weather

☐ SUNNY
☐ CLOUDY
☐ RAINY

Temp: _____

### Mood before Headache:

○ Happy
○ Normal
○ Indifferent
○ Nervous
○ Tired
○ Sad
Other: _____

## Medications & Supplements

_____
_____
_____
_____
_____

## Other Relief Methods:

☐ ICE ☐ RELAX
☐ HEAT ☐ OTHER
☐ BED REST
☐ MASSAGE
☐ LOWER LIGHTS

## Food Intake _____

_____
_____
_____
_____
_____
_____

## Hours of Sleep

_____

## Water Intake

# Notes

Date:      Start Time:      Severity/Intensity

End Time:      ⓪ ① ② ③ ④ ⑤

## Location of headache
○ SINUS   ○CLUSTER   ○TENSION   ○MIGRAINE   ○NECK   ○ TMJ

## Other Symptoms _____

_____

| Triggers | | Weather | Mood before Headache: |
|---|---|---|---|
| ○ Alcohol | ○ Stress at Home | ☐ SUNNY | |
| ○ Caffeine | ○ Stress at Work | ☐ CLOUDY | ○ Happy |
| ○ Hunger | ○ Eyestrain | ☐ RAINY | ○ Normal |
| ○ Tiredness | ○ Weather | Temp: _____ | ○ Indifferent |
| ○ Allergies | ○ PMS | | ○ Nervous |
| ○ Chocolate | ○ Odor | | ○ Tired |
| ○ Other: _____ | | | ○ Sad |

Other: _____

## Medications & Supplements

_____

_____

_____

_____

### Other Relief Methods:
☐ ICE    ☐ RELAX
☐ HEAT   ☐OTHER
☐ BED REST
☐ MASSAGE
☐ LOWER LIGHTS

## Food Intake _____

_____

_____

_____

_____

_____

_____

## Hours of Sleep

## Water Intake
🝙 🝙 🝙 🝙 🝙

🝙 🝙 🝙 🝙 🝙

**Date:**  **Start Time:**  **Severity/Intensity**

**End Time:**  ⓪ ① ② ③ ④ ⑤

## Location of headache

○ SINUS  ○ CLUSTER  ○ TENSION  ○ MIGRAINE  ○ NECK  ○ TMJ

## Other Symptoms _____

_____

| ## Triggers | ## ☁Weather | ## Mood before Headache: |
|---|---|---|

### Triggers

○ Alcohol  ○ Stress at Home
○ Caffeine  ○ Stress at Work
○ Hunger  ○ Eyestrain
○ Tiredness  ○ Weather
○ Allergies  ○ PMS
○ Chocolate  ○ Odor
○ Other: _____

### ☁Weather

☐ SUNNY
☐ CLOUDY
☐ RAINY
Temp: _____

### Mood before Headache:

○ Happy
○ Normal
○ Indifferent
○ Nervous
○ Tired
○ Sad

Other: _____

## 💊 Medications & Supplements

_____
_____
_____
_____
_____

### Other Relief Methods:

☐ ICE  ☐ RELAX
☐ HEAT  ☐ OTHER
☐ BED REST
☐ MASSAGE
☐ LOWER LIGHTS

## 🍳 Food Intake _____

_____
_____
_____
_____
_____
_____

## ☽ Hours of Sleep

_____

## 💧 Water Intake

🍶 🍶 🍶 🍶 🍶

🍶 🍶 🍶 🍶 🍶

## Notes

_____

_____

_____

_____

_____

_____

_____

_____

_____

_____

_____

_____

_____

_____

_____

_____

_____

_____

_____

Date:      Start Time:      Severity/Intensity

End Time:    ( 0 ) ( 1 ) ( 2 ) ( 3 ) ( 4 ) ( 5 )

## Location of headache
○ SINUS ○ CLUSTER ○ TENSION ○ MIGRAINE ○ NECK ○ TMJ

## Other Symptoms _____

_____

| Triggers | Weather | Mood before |
|---|---|---|
| ○ Alcohol ○ Stress at Home | ☐ SUNNY | Headache: |
| ○ Caffeine ○ Stress at Work | ☐ CLOUDY | ○ Happy |
| ○ Hunger ○ Eyestrain | ☐ RAINY | ○ Normal |
| ○ Tiredness ○ Weather | Temp: _____ | ○ Indifferent |
| ○ Allergies ○ PMS | | ○ Nervous |
| ○ Chocolate ○ Odor | | ○ Tired |
| ○ Other: _____ | | ○ Sad |

Other:
_____

## Medications & Supplements

_____
_____
_____
_____
_____

### Other Relief Methods:
☐ ICE     ☐ RELAX
☐ HEAT   ☐ OTHER
☐ BED REST
☐ MASSAGE
☐ LOWER LIGHTS

## Food Intake _____

_____
_____
_____
_____
_____
_____

## Hours of Sleep

_____

## Water Intake

**Date:** 　　　　**Start Time:** 　　　　**Severity/Intensity**

**End Time:** 　　　( 0 ) ( 1 ) ( 2 ) ( 3 ) ( 4 ) ( 5 )

## Location of headache

○ SINUS　○ CLUSTER　○ TENSION　○ MIGRAINE　○ NECK　○ TMJ

## Other Symptoms _____

_____

| Triggers | | ☁ Weather | Mood before |
|---|---|---|---|

### Triggers

- ○ Alcohol
- ○ Caffeine
- ○ Hunger
- ○ Tiredness
- ○ Allergies
- ○ Chocolate
- ○ Other: _____

- ○ Stress at Home
- ○ Stress at Work
- ○ Eyestrain
- ○ Weather
- ○ PMS
- ○ Odor

### ☁ Weather

- ☐ SUNNY
- ☐ CLOUDY
- ☐ RAINY

Temp: _____

### Mood before Headache:

- ○ Happy
- ○ Normal
- ○ Indifferent
- ○ Nervous
- ○ Tired
- ○ Sad

Other: _____

## 💊 Medications & Supplements

_____

_____

_____

_____

_____

## Other Relief Methods:

- ☐ ICE　☐ RELAX
- ☐ HEAT　☐ OTHER
- ☐ BED REST
- ☐ MASSAGE
- ☐ LOWER LIGHTS

## 🍽 Food Intake _____

_____

_____

_____

_____

_____

## ☾ Hours of Sleep

_____

## 💧 Water Intake

🍼 🍼 🍼 🍼 🍼

🍼 🍼 🍼 🍼 🍼

## Notes

# Date:     Start Time:     Severity/Intensity

End Time:    ( 0 ) ( 1 ) ( 2 ) ( 3 ) ( 4 ) ( 5 )

## Location of headache

○ SINUS   ○ CLUSTER   ○ TENSION   ○ MIGRAINE   ○ NECK   ○ TMJ

## Other Symptoms _____

_____

### Triggers

○ Alcohol    ○ Stress at Home
○ Caffeine    ○ Stress at Work
○ Hunger    ○ Eyestrain
○ Tiredness   ○ Weather
○ Allergies    ○ PMS
○ Chocolate   ○ Odor
○ Other: _____

### Weather

☐ SUNNY
☐ CLOUDY
☐ RAINY
Temp: _____

### Mood before Headache:

○ Happy
○ Normal
○ Indifferent
○ Nervous
○ Tired
○ Sad
Other:
_____

## Medications & Supplements

_____
_____
_____
_____
_____

### Other Relief Methods:

☐ ICE    ☐ RELAX
☐ HEAT   ☐ OTHER
☐ BED REST
☐ MASSAGE
☐ LOWER LIGHTS

## Food Intake _____

_____
_____
_____
_____
_____

## Hours of Sleep

_____

## Water Intake

🍶 🍶 🍶 🍶 🍶

🍶 🍶 🍶 🍶 🍶

**Date:**     **Start Time:**     **Severity/Intensity**

**End Time:**     (0) (1) (2) (3) (4) (5)

## Location of headache
○ SINUS   ○ CLUSTER   ○ TENSION    ○ MIGRAINE   ○ NECK   ○ TMJ

## Other Symptoms _____

_____

| ## Triggers | ## ☁ Weather | ## Mood before Headache: |
|---|---|---|
| ○ Alcohol   ○ Stress at Home | ☐ SUNNY | ○ Happy |
| ○ Caffeine   ○ Stress at Work | ☐ CLOUDY | ○ Normal |
| ○ Hunger   ○ Eyestrain | ☐ RAINY | ○ Indifferent |
| ○ Tiredness   ○ Weather | Temp: _____ | ○ Nervous |
| ○ Allergies   ○ PMS | | ○ Tired |
| ○ Chocolate   ○ Odor | | ○ Sad |
| ○ Other: _____ | Other: | |

## 💊 Medications & Supplements

_____

_____

_____

_____

_____

## Other Relief Methods:

☐ ICE    ☐ RELAX
☐ HEAT   ☐ OTHER
☐ BED REST
☐ MASSAGE
☐ LOWER LIGHTS

## 🍳 Food Intake _____

_____

_____

_____

_____

_____

## 🌙 Hours of Sleep

_____

## 💧 Water Intake

🍾 🍾 🍾 🍾 🍾

🍾 🍾 🍾 🍾 🍾

## Notes

Date:     Start Time:     Severity/Intensity

End Time:     ⓪ ① ② ③ ④ ⑤

## Location of headache

○ SINUS   ○ CLUSTER   ○ TENSION   ○ MIGRAINE   ○ NECK   ○ TMJ

## Other Symptoms

---

### Triggers

- ○ Alcohol
- ○ Caffeine
- ○ Hunger
- ○ Tiredness
- ○ Allergies
- ○ Chocolate
- ○ Other:

- ○ Stress at Home
- ○ Stress at Work
- ○ Eyestrain
- ○ Weather
- ○ PMS
- ○ Odor

### Weather

- ☐ SUNNY
- ☐ CLOUDY
- ☐ RAINY

Temp:

### Mood before Headache:

- ○ Happy
- ○ Normal
- ○ Indifferent
- ○ Nervous
- ○ Tired
- ○ Sad

Other:

## Medications & Supplements

_____

_____

_____

_____

_____

### Other Relief Methods:

- ☐ ICE
- ☐ RELAX
- ☐ HEAT
- ☐ OTHER
- ☐ BED REST
- ☐ MASSAGE
- ☐ LOWER LIGHTS

## Food Intake

_____

_____

_____

_____

_____

_____

## Hours of Sleep

## Water Intake

**Date:**      **Start Time:**      **Severity/Intensity**

**End Time:**      ⓪ ① ② ③ ④ ⑤

## Location of headache
○ SINUS   ○ CLUSTER   ○ TENSION   ○ MIGRAINE   ○ NECK   ○ TMJ

## Other Symptoms _____

_____

| Triggers | | ☁ Weather | Mood before Headache: |
|---|---|---|---|
| ○ Alcohol | ○ Stress at Home | ☐ SUNNY | ○ Happy |
| ○ Caffeine | ○ Stress at Work | ☐ CLOUDY | ○ Normal |
| ○ Hunger | ○ Eyestrain | ☐ RAINY | ○ Indifferent |
| ○ Tiredness | ○ Weather | Temp: _____ | ○ Nervous |
| ○ Allergies | ○ PMS | | ○ Tired |
| ○ Chocolate | ○ Odor | | ○ Sad |
| ○ Other: _____ | | | Other: ____ |

## 💊 Medications & Supplements

_____

_____

_____

_____

### Other Relief Methods:
☐ ICE    ☐ RELAX
☐ HEAT   ☐ OTHER
☐ BED REST
☐ MASSAGE
☐ LOWER LIGHTS

## 🍳 Food Intake _____

_____

_____

_____

_____

_____

## 🌙 Hours of Sleep

_____

## 💧 Water Intake

🍼 🍼 🍼 🍼 🍼

🍼 🍼 🍼 🍼 🍼

## Notes

Date:      Start Time:     Severity/Intensity

End Time:     ( 0 ) ( 1 ) ( 2 ) ( 3 ) ( 4 ) ( 5 )

## Location of headache
○ SINUS   ○ CLUSTER   ○ TENSION    ○ MIGRAINE   ○ NECK   ○ TMJ

## Other Symptoms _____

_____

| Triggers | | Weather | Mood before |
|---|---|---|---|

### Triggers
○ Alcohol    ○ Stress at Home
○ Caffeine   ○ Stress at Work
○ Hunger    ○ Eyestrain
○ Tiredness   ○ Weather
○ Allergies   ○ PMS
○ Chocolate   ○ Odor
○ Other: _____

### Weather
☐ SUNNY
☐ CLOUDY
☐ RAINY
Temp: _____

### Mood before Headache:
○ Happy
○ Normal
○ Indifferent
○ Nervous
○ Tired
○ Sad
Other:
_____

## Medications & Supplements

_____

_____

_____

_____

_____

### Other Relief Methods:
☐ ICE     ☐ RELAX
☐ HEAT   ☐ OTHER
☐ BED REST
☐ MASSAGE
☐ LOWER LIGHTS

## Food Intake _____

_____

_____

_____

_____

_____

### Hours of Sleep

_____

### Water Intake

# Notes

Date: Start Time: Severity/Intensity

End Time: (0) (1) (2) (3) (4) (5)

## Location of headache
○ SINUS ○ CLUSTER ○ TENSION ○ MIGRAINE ○ NECK ○ TMJ

## Other Symptoms _____

_____

| Triggers | Weather | Mood before Headache: |
|---|---|---|

○ Alcohol ○ Stress at Home ☐ SUNNY

○ Caffeine ○ Stress at Work ☐ CLOUDY ○ Happy

○ Hunger ○ Eyestrain ☐ RAINY ○ Normal

○ Tiredness ○ Weather Temp: _____ ○ Indifferent

○ Allergies ○ PMS ○ Nervous

○ Chocolate ○ Odor ○ Tired

○ Other: _____ ○ Sad

Other: _____

## Medications & Supplements

_____

_____

_____

_____

_____

### Other Relief Methods:
☐ ICE ☐ RELAX
☐ HEAT ☐ OTHER
☐ BED REST
☐ MASSAGE
☐ LOWER LIGHTS

## Food Intake _____

## Hours of Sleep
_____

_____

_____

## Water Intake

_____

_____

_____

_____

_____

Date:      Start Time:      Severity/Intensity

End Time:     ⓪ ① ② ③ ④ ⑤

## Location of headache

○ SINUS ○ CLUSTER ○ TENSION ○ MIGRAINE ○ NECK ○ TMJ

## Other Symptoms _____

_____

| Triggers | | Weather | Mood before |
|---|---|---|---|

○ Alcohol    ○ Stress at Home    ☐ SUNNY    **Headache:**

○ Caffeine    ○ Stress at Work    ☐ CLOUDY    ○ Happy

○ Hunger    ○ Eyestrain    ☐ RAINY    ○ Normal

○ Tiredness    ○ Weather    Temp: _____    ○ Indifferent

○ Allergies    ○ PMS        ○ Nervous

○ Chocolate    ○ Odor        ○ Tired

○ Other: _____        ○ Sad

                        Other:

                        _____

## Medications & Supplements

_____

_____

_____

_____

_____

### Other Relief Methods:

☐ ICE     ☐ RELAX

☐ HEAT    ☐ OTHER

☐ BED REST

☐ MASSAGE

☐ LOWER LIGHTS

## Food Intake _____

_____

_____

_____

_____

_____

_____

### Hours of Sleep

_____

## Water Intake

🍾 🍾 🍾 🍾 🍾

🍾 🍾 🍾 🍾 🍾

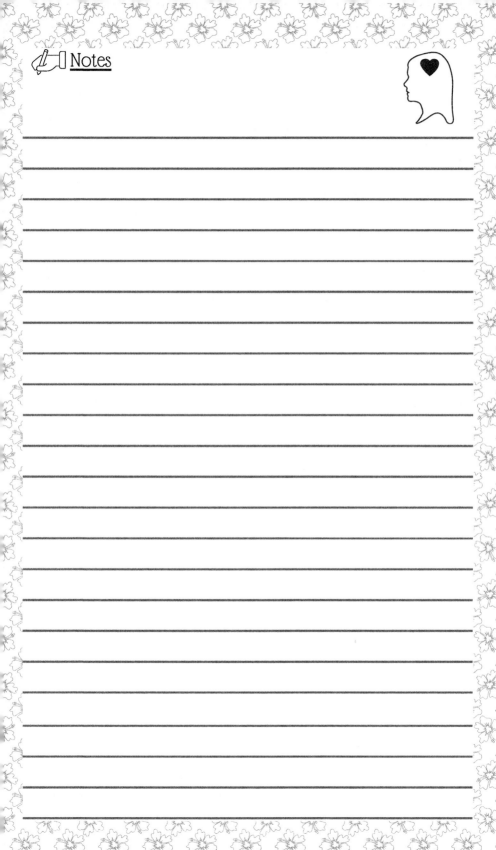

## Notes

_____

_____

_____

_____

_____

_____

_____

_____

_____

_____

_____

_____

_____

_____

_____

_____

_____

_____

Date:                 Start Time:              Severity/Intensity

                      End Time:          ⓪  ①  ②  ③  ④  ⑤

## Location of headache
○ SINUS  ○ CLUSTER  ○ TENSION   ○ MIGRAINE  ○ NECK  ○ TMJ

## Other Symptoms _____

_____

### Triggers            ☁ Weather          Mood before
○ Alcohol   ○ Stress at Home    ☐ SUNNY        Headache:
○ Caffeine  ○ Stress at Work    ☐ CLOUDY    ○  Happy
○ Hunger    ○ Eyestrain         ☐ RAINY     ○  Normal
○ Tiredness ○ Weather       Temp: _____    ○  Indifferent
○ Allergies ○ PMS                            ○  Nervous
○ Chocolate ○ Odor                           ○  Tired
○ Other:                                     ○  Sad
        _____          Other:
                                         _____

### 💊 Medications & Supplements        Other Relief
                                          Methods:
_____    ☐ ICE    ☐ RELAX
_____    ☐ HEAT   ☐ OTHER
_____    ☐ BED REST
_____    ☐ MASSAGE
_____    ☐ LOWER LIGHTS

### 🍳 Food Intake _____     🌙 Hours of Sleep

_____       _____

_____    💧 Water Intake
_____
_____    🍶 🍶 🍶 🍶 🍶
_____
_____    🍶 🍶 🍶 🍶 🍶

# Notes

Date:      Start Time:      Severity/Intensity

End Time:    (0) (1) (2) (3) (4) (5)

## Location of headache

O SINUS   OCLUSTER   OTENSION    OMIGRAINE   ONECK   O TMJ

## Other Symptoms _____

_____

### Triggers      Weather     Mood before

| Triggers | | Weather | Headache: |
|---|---|---|---|
| O Alcohol | O Stress at Home | ☐ SUNNY | |
| O Caffeine | O Stress at Work | ☐ CLOUDY | O Happy |
| O Hunger | O Eyestrain | ☐ RAINY | O Normal |
| O Tiredness | O Weather | Temp: ____ | O Indifferent |
| O Allergies | O PMS | | O Nervous |
| O Chocolate | O Odor | | O Tired |
| O Other: ____ | | | O Sad |

Other:
_____

## Medications & Supplements

_____

_____

_____

_____

_____

## Other Relief Methods:

☐ ICE    ☐ RELAX
☐ HEAT   ☐ OTHER
☐ BED REST
☐ MASSAGE
☐ LOWER LIGHTS

## Food Intake _____

_____

_____

_____

_____

_____

## Hours of Sleep

_____

## Water Intake

🍶 🍶 🍶 🍶 🍶

🍶 🍶 🍶 🍶 🍶

# Notes

Date: Start Time: Severity/Intensity

End Time: (0) (1) (2) (3) (4) (5)

## Location of headache
○ SINUS  ○ CLUSTER  ○ TENSION  ○ MIGRAINE  ○ NECK  ○ TMJ

## Other Symptoms _____

_____

| ## Triggers | | ## Weather | ## Mood before Headache: |
|---|---|---|---|
| ○ Alcohol | ○ Stress at Home | ☐ SUNNY | |
| ○ Caffeine | ○ Stress at Work | ☐ CLOUDY | ○ Happy |
| ○ Hunger | ○ Eyestrain | ☐ RAINY | ○ Normal |
| ○ Tiredness | ○ Weather | Temp: _____ | ○ Indifferent |
| ○ Allergies | ○ PMS | | ○ Nervous |
| ○ Chocolate | ○ Odor | | ○ Tired |
| ○ Other: | | | ○ Sad |

Other:
_____

## Medications & Supplements

_____

_____

_____

_____

_____

### Other Relief Methods:
☐ ICE  ☐ RELAX
☐ HEAT  ☐ OTHER
☐ BED REST
☐ MASSAGE
☐ LOWER LIGHTS

## Food Intake _____

_____

_____

_____

_____

_____

## Hours of Sleep

_____

## Water Intake

**Date:** **Start Time:** **Severity/Intensity**

**End Time:** ⓪ ① ② ③ ④ ⑤

## Location of headache
○ SINUS  ○ CLUSTER  ○ TENSION  ○ MIGRAINE  ○ NECK  ○ TMJ

## Other Symptoms _____

_____

### Triggers
○ Alcohol  ○ Stress at Home
○ Caffeine  ○ Stress at Work
○ Hunger  ○ Eyestrain
○ Tiredness  ○ Weather
○ Allergies  ○ PMS
○ Chocolate  ○ Odor
○ Other: _____

### ☁ Weather
☐ SUNNY
☐ CLOUDY
☐ RAINY
Temp: _____

### Mood before Headache:
○ Happy
○ Normal
○ Indifferent
○ Nervous
○ Tired
○ Sad
Other:
_____

### 💊 Medications & Supplements
_____
_____
_____
_____

### Other Relief Methods:
☐ ICE       ☐ RELAX
☐ HEAT    ☐ OTHER
☐ BED REST
☐ MASSAGE
☐ LOWER LIGHTS

### 🍽 Food Intake _____
_____
_____
_____
_____
_____

### ☽ Hours of Sleep
_____

### 💧 Water Intake
🍶 🍶 🍶 🍶 🍶

🍶 🍶 🍶 🍶 🍶

**Date:**       **Start Time:**       **Severity/Intensity**

             **End Time:**       ( 0 )  ( 1 )  ( 2 )  ( 3 )  ( 4 )  ( 5 )

## Location of headache
○ SINUS  ○ CLUSTER  ○ TENSION   ○ MIGRAINE  ○ NECK  ○ TMJ

## Other Symptoms _____

_____

| ## Triggers | ## ☁Weather | ## Mood before |
|---|---|---|

### Triggers

○ Alcohol    ○ Stress at Home
○ Caffeine   ○ Stress at Work
○ Hunger     ○ Eyestrain
○ Tiredness  ○ Weather
○ Allergies  ○ PMS
○ Chocolate  ○ Odor
○ Other: _____

### ☁ Weather

☐ SUNNY
☐ CLOUDY
☐ RAINY

Temp: _____

### Mood before Headache:

○  Happy
○  Normal
○  Indifferent
○  Nervous
○  Tired
○  Sad

Other: _____

## 💊 Medications & Supplements

_____
_____
_____
_____
_____

### Other Relief Methods:

☐ ICE     ☐ RELAX
☐ HEAT   ☐ OTHER
☐ BED REST
☐ MASSAGE
☐ LOWER LIGHTS

## 🍳 Food Intake _____

_____
_____
_____
_____
_____

### ☾ Hours of Sleep

_____

### ◊ Water Intake

🍶 🍶 🍶 🍶 🍶

🍶 🍶 🍶 🍶 🍶

Date:     Start Time:     Severity/Intensity

End Time:     (0) (1) (2) (3) (4) (5)

## Location of headache
○ SINUS ○ CLUSTER ○ TENSION ○ MIGRAINE ○ NECK ○ TMJ

## Other Symptoms _____

_____

### Triggers
○ Alcohol    ○ Stress at Home
○ Caffeine    ○ Stress at Work
○ Hunger    ○ Eyestrain
○ Tiredness    ○ Weather
○ Allergies    ○ PMS
○ Chocolate    ○ Odor
○ Other: _____

### Weather
☐ SUNNY
☐ CLOUDY
☐ RAINY
Temp: _____

### Mood before Headache:
○ Happy
○ Normal
○ Indifferent
○ Nervous
○ Tired
○ Sad
Other: _____

## Medications & Supplements
_____
_____
_____
_____
_____
_____

### Other Relief Methods:
☐ ICE    ☐ RELAX
☐ HEAT    ☐ OTHER
☐ BED REST
☐ MASSAGE
☐ LOWER LIGHTS

## Food Intake _____
_____
_____
_____
_____
_____

### Hours of Sleep
_____

### Water Intake

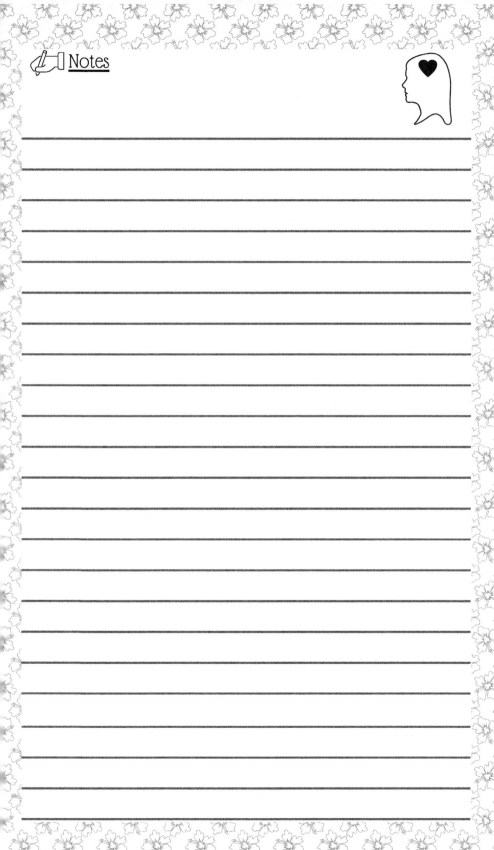

## Notes

**Date:** _____ **Start Time:** _____

**End Time:** _____

**Severity/Intensity**

(0) (1) (2) (3) (4) (5)

## Location of headache

○ SINUS  ○ CLUSTER  ○ TENSION  ○ MIGRAINE  ○ NECK  ○ TMJ

## Other Symptoms _____

_____

## Triggers

○ Alcohol    ○ Stress at Home
○ Caffeine   ○ Stress at Work
○ Hunger     ○ Eyestrain
○ Tiredness  ○ Weather
○ Allergies  ○ PMS
○ Chocolate  ○ Odor
○ Other: _____

## Weather

☐ SUNNY
☐ CLOUDY
☐ RAINY

Temp: _____

## Mood before Headache:

○ Happy
○ Normal
○ Indifferent
○ Nervous
○ Tired
○ Sad

Other: _____

## Medications & Supplements

_____
_____
_____
_____
_____

## Other Relief Methods:

☐ ICE      ☐ RELAX
☐ HEAT     ☐ OTHER
☐ BED REST
☐ MASSAGE
☐ LOWER LIGHTS

## Food Intake _____

_____
_____
_____
_____
_____

## Hours of Sleep

_____

## Water Intake

🍶 🍶 🍶 🍶 🍶

🍶 🍶 🍶 🍶 🍶

# Notes

_____

_____

_____

_____

_____

_____

_____

_____

_____

_____

_____

_____

_____

_____

_____

_____

_____

_____

**Date:** **Start Time:** **Severity/Intensity**

**End Time:** (0) (1) (2) (3) (4) (5)

## Location of headache

○ SINUS  ○ CLUSTER  ○ TENSION  ○ MIGRAINE  ○ NECK  ○ TMJ

## Other Symptoms _____

_____

### Triggers

○ Alcohol    ○ Stress at Home
○ Caffeine   ○ Stress at Work
○ Hunger     ○ Eyestrain
○ Tiredness  ○ Weather
○ Allergies  ○ PMS
○ Chocolate  ○ Odor
○ Other: _____

### ☁ Weather

☐ SUNNY
☐ CLOUDY
☐ RAINY
Temp: _____

### Mood before Headache:

○ Happy
○ Normal
○ Indifferent
○ Nervous
○ Tired
○ Sad
Other:
_____

## 💊 Medications & Supplements

_____

_____

_____

_____

_____

### Other Relief Methods:

☐ ICE     ☐ RELAX
☐ HEAT    ☐ OTHER
☐ BED REST
☐ MASSAGE
☐ LOWER LIGHTS

## 🍳 Food Intake _____

_____

_____

_____

_____

_____

_____

### ☽ Hours of Sleep

_____

### ○ Water Intake

🍶 🍶 🍶 🍶 🍶

🍶 🍶 🍶 🍶 🍶

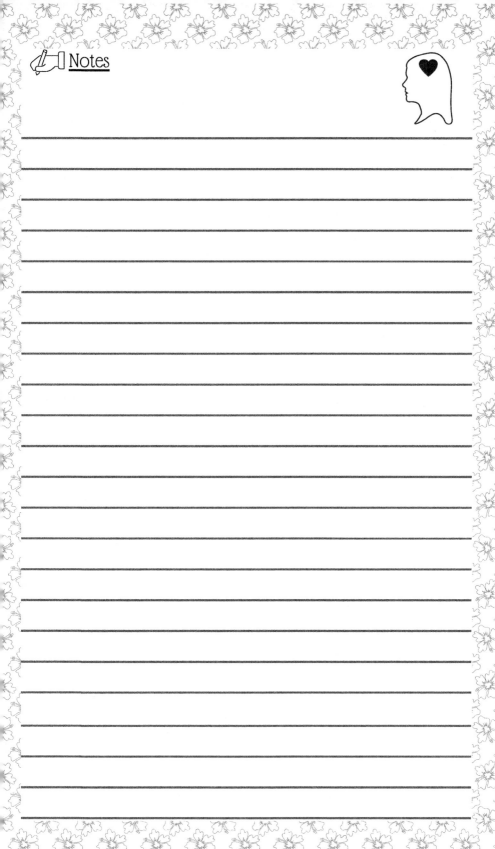

## Notes

**Date:** **Start Time:** **Severity/Intensity**

**End Time:** (0) (1) (2) (3) (4) (5)

## Location of headache
○ SINUS  ○ CLUSTER  ○ TENSION  ○ MIGRAINE  ○ NECK  ○ TMJ

## Other Symptoms _____

_____

| Triggers | | Weather | Mood before Headache: |
|---|---|---|---|
| ○ Alcohol | ○ Stress at Home | ☐ SUNNY | ○ Happy |
| ○ Caffeine | ○ Stress at Work | ☐ CLOUDY | ○ Normal |
| ○ Hunger | ○ Eyestrain | ☐ RAINY | ○ Indifferent |
| ○ Tiredness | ○ Weather | Temp: _____ | ○ Nervous |
| ○ Allergies | ○ PMS | | ○ Tired |
| ○ Chocolate | ○ Odor | | ○ Sad |
| ○ Other: _____ | | | Other: |

_____

## Medications & Supplements

### Other Relief Methods:

_____ ☐ ICE  ☐ RELAX

_____ ☐ HEAT  ☐ OTHER

_____ ☐ BED REST

_____ ☐ MASSAGE

_____ ☐ LOWER LIGHTS

## Food Intake _____

## Hours of Sleep

_____

_____

_____ ## Water Intake

_____

_____

_____

Date: Start Time: **Severity/Intensity**

End Time: ( 0 ) ( 1 ) ( 2 ) ( 3 ) ( 4 ) ( 5 )

## Location of headache

○ SINUS  ○ CLUSTER  ○ TENSION  ○ MIGRAINE  ○ NECK  ○ TMJ

## Other Symptoms _____

_____

### Triggers

○ Alcohol  ○ Stress at Home
○ Caffeine  ○ Stress at Work
○ Hunger  ○ Eyestrain
○ Tiredness  ○ Weather
○ Allergies  ○ PMS
○ Chocolate  ○ Odor
○ Other: _____

### Weather

☐ SUNNY
☐ CLOUDY
☐ RAINY

Temp: _____

### Mood before Headache:

○ Happy
○ Normal
○ Indifferent
○ Nervous
○ Tired
○ Sad

Other: _____

## Medications & Supplements

_____
_____
_____
_____
_____

### Other Relief Methods:

☐ ICE  ☐ RELAX
☐ HEAT  ☐ OTHER
☐ BED REST
☐ MASSAGE
☐ LOWER LIGHTS

## Food Intake _____

_____
_____
_____
_____
_____
_____

## Hours of Sleep

_____

## Water Intake

# Notes

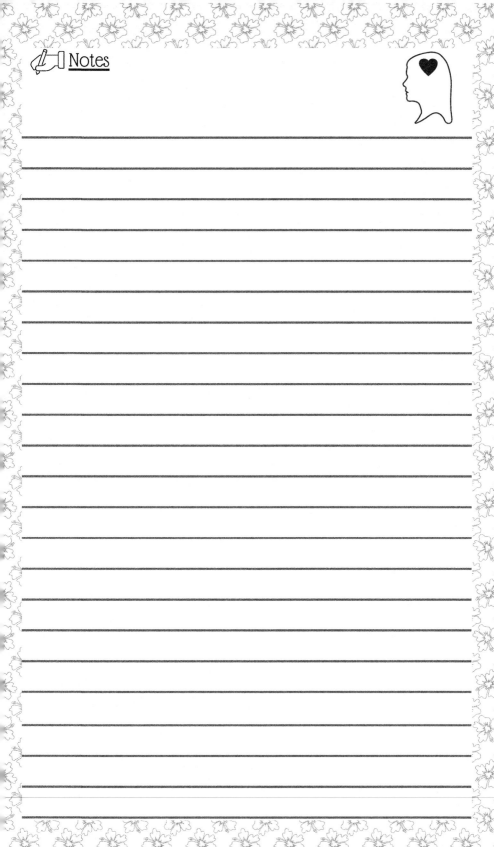

**Date:**     **Start Time:**     **Severity/Intensity**

**End Time:**    (0) (1) (2) (3) (4) (5)

## Location of headache

○ SINUS   ○ CLUSTER   ○ TENSION    ○ MIGRAINE   ○ NECK   ○ TMJ

## Other Symptoms _____

_____

### Triggers       Weather     Mood before

| | | | Headache: |
|---|---|---|---|
| ○ Alcohol | ○ Stress at Home | ☐ SUNNY | |
| ○ Caffeine | ○ Stress at Work | ☐ CLOUDY | ○ Happy |
| ○ Hunger | ○ Eyestrain | ☐ RAINY | ○ Normal |
| ○ Tiredness | ○ Weather | Temp: _____ | ○ Indifferent |
| ○ Allergies | ○ PMS | | ○ Nervous |
| ○ Chocolate | ○ Odor | | ○ Tired |
| ○ Other: | | | ○ Sad |

_____    Other: _____

## Medications & Supplements

_____

_____

_____

_____

_____

### Other Relief Methods:

☐ ICE    ☐ RELAX
☐ HEAT   ☐ OTHER
☐ BED REST
☐ MASSAGE
☐ LOWER LIGHTS

## Food Intake _____

_____

_____

_____

_____

_____

_____

### Hours of Sleep

_____

### Water Intake

🍶 🍶 🍶 🍶 🍶

🍶 🍶 🍶 🍶 🍶

Date:      Start Time:      Severity/Intensity

End Time:    ( 0 ) ( 1 ) ( 2 ) ( 3 ) ( 4 ) ( 5 )

## Location of headache

○ SINUS   ○ CLUSTER   ○ TENSION    ○ MIGRAINE   ○ NECK   ○ TMJ

## Other Symptoms _____

_____

| Triggers | | Weather | Mood before |
|---|---|---|---|
| ○ Alcohol | ○ Stress at Home | ☐ SUNNY | Headache: |
| ○ Caffeine | ○ Stress at Work | ☐ CLOUDY | ○ Happy |
| ○ Hunger | ○ Eyestrain | ☐ RAINY | ○ Normal |
| ○ Tiredness | ○ Weather | Temp: _____ | ○ Indifferent |
| ○ Allergies | ○ PMS | | ○ Nervous |
| ○ Chocolate | ○ Odor | | ○ Tired |
| ○ Other: _____ | | | ○ Sad |
| | | | Other: |

_____

## Medications & Supplements

_____

_____

_____

_____

_____

### Other Relief Methods:

☐ ICE    ☐ RELAX
☐ HEAT   ☐ OTHER
☐ BED REST
☐ MASSAGE
☐ LOWER LIGHTS

## Food Intake _____

_____

## Hours of Sleep

_____

## Water Intake

_____

_____

_____

_____

_____

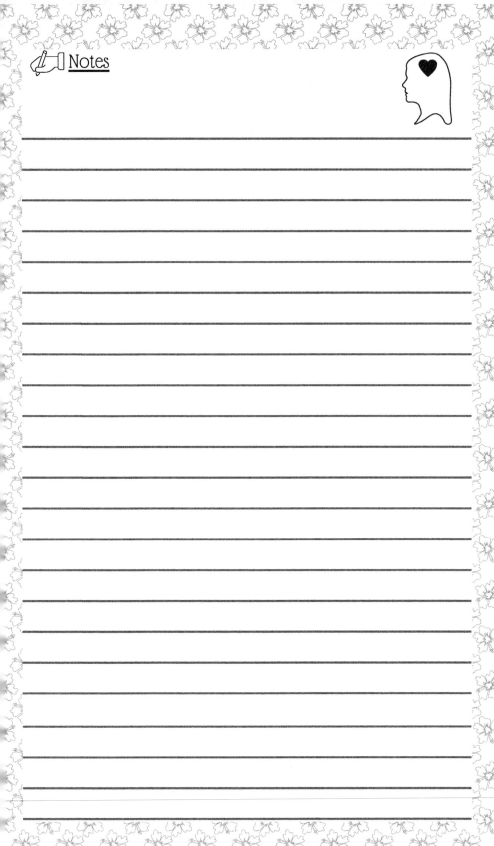

## Notes

**Date:**     **Start Time:**     **Severity/Intensity**

**End Time:**    (0) (1) (2) (3) (4) (5)

## Location of headache
○ SINUS ○ CLUSTER ○ TENSION ○ MIGRAINE ○ NECK ○ TMJ

## Other Symptoms _____

_____

| Triggers | Weather | Mood before Headache: |
|---|---|---|
| ○ Alcohol   ○ Stress at Home | ☐ SUNNY | ○ Happy |
| ○ Caffeine   ○ Stress at Work | ☐ CLOUDY | ○ Normal |
| ○ Hunger   ○ Eyestrain | ☐ RAINY | ○ Indifferent |
| ○ Tiredness   ○ Weather | Temp: _____ | ○ Nervous |
| ○ Allergies   ○ PMS | | ○ Tired |
| ○ Chocolate   ○ Odor | | ○ Sad |
| ○ Other: _____ | | Other: |

_____

## Medications & Supplements

_____

_____

_____

_____

_____

### Other Relief Methods:
☐ ICE    ☐ RELAX
☐ HEAT   ☐ OTHER
☐ BED REST
☐ MASSAGE
☐ LOWER LIGHTS

## Food Intake _____

_____

_____

_____

_____

_____

## ☾ Hours of Sleep

_____

## ○ Water Intake
🍼 🍼 🍼 🍼 🍼

🍼 🍼 🍼 🍼 🍼

# Notes

Date:     Start Time:     Severity/Intensity

End Time:     ( 0 ) ( 1 ) ( 2 ) ( 3 ) ( 4 ) ( 5 )

## Location of headache

○ SINUS ○ CLUSTER ○ TENSION ○ MIGRAINE ○ NECK ○ TMJ

## Other Symptoms _____

_____

### Triggers
- ○ Alcohol   ○ Stress at Home
- ○ Caffeine   ○ Stress at Work
- ○ Hunger   ○ Eyestrain
- ○ Tiredness   ○ Weather
- ○ Allergies   ○ PMS
- ○ Chocolate   ○ Odor
- ○ Other: _____

### ☁ Weather
- ☐ SUNNY
- ☐ CLOUDY
- ☐ RAINY

Temp: _____

### Mood before Headache:
- ○ Happy
- ○ Normal
- ○ Indifferent
- ○ Nervous
- ○ Tired
- ○ Sad

Other:
_____

## Medications & Supplements

_____

_____

_____

_____

_____

### Other Relief Methods:
- ☐ ICE    ☐ RELAX
- ☐ HEAT   ☐ OTHER
- ☐ BED REST
- ☐ MASSAGE
- ☐ LOWER LIGHTS

## Food Intake _____

_____

_____

_____

_____

_____

### ☾ Hours of Sleep

_____

### ○ Water Intake

🍶 🍶 🍶 🍶 🍶

🍶 🍶 🍶 🍶 🍶

**Date:**      **Start Time:**      **Severity/Intensity**

**End Time:**      ⓪ ① ② ③ ④ ⑤

## Location of headache

○ SINUS   ○ CLUSTER   ○ TENSION   ○ MIGRAINE   ○ NECK   ○ TMJ

## Other Symptoms _____

_____

### Triggers

○ Alcohol    ○ Stress at Home
○ Caffeine    ○ Stress at Work
○ Hunger    ○ Eyestrain
○ Tiredness    ○ Weather
○ Allergies    ○ PMS
○ Chocolate    ○ Odor
○ Other: _____

### Weather

☐ SUNNY
☐ CLOUDY
☐ RAINY
Temp: _____

### Mood before Headache:

○ Happy
○ Normal
○ Indifferent
○ Nervous
○ Tired
○ Sad
Other: _____

### Medications & Supplements

_____
_____
_____
_____
_____

### Other Relief Methods:

☐ ICE    ☐ RELAX
☐ HEAT    ☐ OTHER
☐ BED REST
☐ MASSAGE
☐ LOWER LIGHTS

### Food Intake _____

_____
_____
_____
_____
_____

### Hours of Sleep

_____

### Water Intake

🍶 🍶 🍶 🍶 🍶

🍶 🍶 🍶 🍶 🍶

# ✍ <u>Notes</u>

**Date:**     **Start Time:**     **Severity/Intensity**

**End Time:**     ⓪ ① ② ③ ④ ⑤

## Location of headache

○ SINUS   ○ CLUSTER   ○ TENSION    ○ MIGRAINE   ○ NECK   ○ TMJ

## Other Symptoms _____

_____

### Triggers

- ○ Alcohol
- ○ Caffeine
- ○ Hunger
- ○ Tiredness
- ○ Allergies
- ○ Chocolate
- ○ Other: _____

- ○ Stress at Home
- ○ Stress at Work
- ○ Eyestrain
- ○ Weather
- ○ PMS
- ○ Odor

### ☁ Weather

- ☐ SUNNY
- ☐ CLOUDY
- ☐ RAINY

Temp: _____

### Mood before Headache:

- ○ Happy
- ○ Normal
- ○ Indifferent
- ○ Nervous
- ○ Tired
- ○ Sad

Other: _____

## ⊂⊃ Medications & Supplements

_____

_____

_____

_____

_____

### Other Relief Methods:

- ☐ ICE    ☐ RELAX
- ☐ HEAT   ☐ OTHER
- ☐ BED REST
- ☐ MASSAGE
- ☐ LOWER LIGHTS

## 🍳 Food Intake _____

_____

_____

_____

_____

_____

### ☽ Hours of Sleep

_____

### ◊ Water Intake

🍼 🍼 🍼 🍼 🍼

🍼 🍼 🍼 🍼 🍼

# ✍️ <u>Notes</u>

**Date:** _____  **Start Time:** _____

**End Time:** _____

## Severity/Intensity

( 0 )  ( 1 )  ( 2 )  ( 3 )  ( 4 )  ( 5 )

## Location of headache

○ SINUS  ○ CLUSTER  ○ TENSION  ○ MIGRAINE  ○ NECK  ○ TMJ

## Other Symptoms _____

_____

### Triggers

○ Alcohol     ○ Stress at Home
○ Caffeine    ○ Stress at Work
○ Hunger      ○ Eyestrain
○ Tiredness   ○ Weather
○ Allergies   ○ PMS
○ Chocolate   ○ Odor
○ Other: _____

### ☁ Weather

☐ SUNNY
☐ CLOUDY
☐ RAINY

Temp: _____

### Mood before Headache:

○ Happy
○ Normal
○ Indifferent
○ Nervous
○ Tired
○ Sad

Other: _____

## 💊 Medications & Supplements

_____
_____
_____
_____
_____

## Other Relief Methods:

☐ ICE       ☐ RELAX
☐ HEAT      ☐ OTHER
☐ BED REST
☐ MASSAGE
☐ LOWER LIGHTS

## 🍽 Food Intake _____

_____
_____
_____
_____
_____

## ☾ Hours of Sleep

_____

## ○ Water Intake

🍶 🍶 🍶 🍶 🍶

🍶 🍶 🍶 🍶 🍶

## Notes

Date:      Start Time:      Severity/Intensity

End Time:    ⓪ ① ② ③ ④ ⑤

## Location of headache
○ SINUS ○ CLUSTER ○ TENSION ○ MIGRAINE ○ NECK ○ TMJ

## Other Symptoms _____

_____

| Triggers | | Weather | Mood before Headache: |
|---|---|---|---|
| ○ Alcohol | ○ Stress at Home | ☐ SUNNY | |
| ○ Caffeine | ○ Stress at Work | ☐ CLOUDY | ○ Happy |
| ○ Hunger | ○ Eyestrain | ☐ RAINY | ○ Normal |
| ○ Tiredness | ○ Weather | Temp: | ○ Indifferent |
| ○ Allergies | ○ PMS | | ○ Nervous |
| ○ Chocolate | ○ Odor | | ○ Tired |
| ○ Other: | | | ○ Sad |

Other:
_____

## Medications & Supplements

_____

_____

_____

_____

_____

### Other Relief Methods:
☐ ICE    ☐ RELAX
☐ HEAT ☐ OTHER
☐ BED REST
☐ MASSAGE
☐ LOWER LIGHTS

## Food Intake _____

_____

_____

_____

_____

_____

## Hours of Sleep

_____

## Water Intake

🍶 🍶 🍶 🍶 🍶

🍶 🍶 🍶 🍶 🍶

Notes

Date:      Start Time:      Severity/Intensity

End Time:    (0) (1) (2) (3) (4) (5)

## Location of headache

○ SINUS   ○ CLUSTER   ○ TENSION   ○ MIGRAINE   ○ NECK   ○ TMJ

## Other Symptoms _____

| Triggers | | Weather | Mood before Headache: |
|---|---|---|---|
| ○ Alcohol | ○ Stress at Home | ☐ SUNNY | |
| ○ Caffeine | ○ Stress at Work | ☐ CLOUDY | ○ Happy |
| ○ Hunger | ○ Eyestrain | ☐ RAINY | ○ Normal |
| ○ Tiredness | ○ Weather | Temp: _____ | ○ Indifferent |
| ○ Allergies | ○ PMS | | ○ Nervous |
| ○ Chocolate | ○ Odor | | ○ Tired |
| ○ Other: | | | ○ Sad |

Other: _____

## Medications & Supplements

_____

_____

_____

_____

## Other Relief Methods:

☐ ICE     ☐ RELAX
☐ HEAT    ☐ OTHER
☐ BED REST
☐ MASSAGE
☐ LOWER LIGHTS

## Food Intake _____

_____

_____

_____

_____

_____

_____

## Hours of Sleep

_____

## Water Intake

Date: _____  Start Time: _____  Severity/Intensity

End Time: _____  (0) (1) (2) (3) (4) (5)

## Location of headache

○ SINUS  ○ CLUSTER  ○ TENSION  ○ MIGRAINE  ○ NECK  ○ TMJ

## Other Symptoms _____

| Triggers | Weather | Mood before |
|---|---|---|

### Triggers
- ○ Alcohol
- ○ Caffeine
- ○ Hunger
- ○ Tiredness
- ○ Allergies
- ○ Chocolate
- ○ Other: _____

- ○ Stress at Home
- ○ Stress at Work
- ○ Eyestrain
- ○ Weather
- ○ PMS
- ○ Odor

### Weather
- ☐ SUNNY
- ☐ CLOUDY
- ☐ RAINY

Temp: _____

### Mood before Headache:
- ○ Happy
- ○ Normal
- ○ Indifferent
- ○ Nervous
- ○ Tired
- ○ Sad

Other:

## Medications & Supplements

_____
_____
_____
_____
_____

### Other Relief Methods:
- ☐ ICE   ☐ RELAX
- ☐ HEAT  ☐ OTHER
- ☐ BED REST
- ☐ MASSAGE
- ☐ LOWER LIGHTS

## Food Intake _____

_____
_____
_____
_____
_____
_____

### Hours of Sleep

_____

### Water Intake

# Notes

# Date:      Start Time:      Severity/Intensity

End Time:    (0) (1) (2) (3) (4) (5)

## Location of headache
○ SINUS   ○ CLUSTER   ○ TENSION   ○ MIGRAINE   ○ NECK   ○ TMJ

## Other Symptoms _____

### Triggers
○ Alcohol   ○ Stress at Home
○ Caffeine   ○ Stress at Work
○ Hunger   ○ Eyestrain
○ Tiredness   ○ Weather
○ Allergies   ○ PMS
○ Chocolate   ○ Odor
○ Other: _____

### ☁Weather
☐ SUNNY
☐ CLOUDY
☐ RAINY
Temp: _____

### Mood before Headache:
○ Happy
○ Normal
○ Indifferent
○ Nervous
○ Tired
○ Sad
Other:
_____

## 💊 Medications & Supplements
_____
_____
_____
_____
_____

### Other Relief Methods:
☐ ICE    ☐ RELAX
☐ HEAT   ☐ OTHER
☐ BED REST
☐ MASSAGE
☐ LOWER LIGHTS

## Food Intake _____

## 🌙 Hours of Sleep
_____
_____

### 💧 Water Intake
🍶 🍶 🍶 🍶 🍶

🍶 🍶 🍶 🍶 🍶
_____
_____

# Notes

Date:      Start Time:      Severity/Intensity

End Time:    ⓪ ① ② ③ ④ ⑤

## Location of headache
○ SINUS   ○ CLUSTER   ○ TENSION   ○ MIGRAINE   ○ NECK   ○ TMJ

## Other Symptoms _____

---

| Triggers | | Weather | Mood before |
|---|---|---|---|
| ○ Alcohol | ○ Stress at Home | ☐ SUNNY | Headache: |
| ○ Caffeine | ○ Stress at Work | ☐ CLOUDY | ○ Happy |
| ○ Hunger | ○ Eyestrain | ☐ RAINY | ○ Normal |
| ○ Tiredness | ○ Weather | Temp: _____ | ○ Indifferent |
| ○ Allergies | ○ PMS | | ○ Nervous |
| ○ Chocolate | ○ Odor | | ○ Tired |
| ○ Other: _____ | | | ○ Sad |

Other:

## Medications & Supplements

_____

_____

_____

_____

_____

### Other Relief Methods:

☐ ICE    ☐ RELAX
☐ HEAT   ☐ OTHER
☐ BED REST
☐ MASSAGE
☐ LOWER LIGHTS

## Food Intake _____

_____

_____

_____

_____

_____

## Hours of Sleep

_____

## Water Intake

# Notes

**Date:** **Start Time:** **Severity/Intensity**

**End Time:** ( 0 ) ( 1 ) ( 2 ) ( 3 ) ( 4 ) ( 5 )

## Location of headache

○ SINUS  ○ CLUSTER  ○ TENSION  ○ MIGRAINE  ○ NECK  ○ TMJ

## Other Symptoms _____

_____

### Triggers
- ○ Alcohol
- ○ Caffeine
- ○ Hunger
- ○ Tiredness
- ○ Allergies
- ○ Chocolate
- ○ Other: _____

- ○ Stress at Home
- ○ Stress at Work
- ○ Eyestrain
- ○ Weather
- ○ PMS
- ○ Odor

### ☁Weather
- ☐ SUNNY
- ☐ CLOUDY
- ☐ RAINY

Temp: _____

### Mood before Headache:
- ○ Happy
- ○ Normal
- ○ Indifferent
- ○ Nervous
- ○ Tired
- ○ Sad

Other: _____

## 💊 Medications & Supplements

_____

_____

_____

_____

_____

### Other Relief Methods:
- ☐ ICE    ☐ RELAX
- ☐ HEAT   ☐ OTHER
- ☐ BED REST
- ☐ MASSAGE
- ☐ LOWER LIGHTS

## 🍽 Food Intake _____

_____

_____

_____

_____

_____

## 🌙 Hours of Sleep

_____

## 💧 Water Intake

🍶 🍶 🍶 🍶 🍶

🍶 🍶 🍶 🍶 🍶

## Notes

Date:      Start Time:      Severity/Intensity

End Time:     ( 0 ) ( 1 ) ( 2 ) ( 3 ) ( 4 ) ( 5 )

## Location of headache
○ SINUS ○ CLUSTER ○ TENSION ○ MIGRAINE ○ NECK ○ TMJ

## Other Symptoms _____

### Triggers
○ Alcohol ○ Stress at Home
○ Caffeine ○ Stress at Work
○ Hunger ○ Eyestrain
○ Tiredness ○ Weather
○ Allergies ○ PMS
○ Chocolate ○ Odor
○ Other: _____

### Weather
☐ SUNNY
☐ CLOUDY
☐ RAINY
Temp: _____

### Mood before Headache:
○ Happy
○ Normal
○ Indifferent
○ Nervous
○ Tired
○ Sad

Other: _____

## Medications & Supplements

_____
_____
_____
_____

### Other Relief Methods:
☐ ICE    ☐ RELAX
☐ HEAT ☐ OTHER
☐ BED REST
☐ MASSAGE
☐ LOWER LIGHTS

## Food Intake _____

_____
_____
_____
_____
_____
_____

## Hours of Sleep
_____

## Water Intake

# Notes

**Date:** _____ **Start Time:** _____ **Severity/Intensity**

**End Time:** _____ ⓪ ① ② ③ ④ ⑤

## Location of headache

○ SINUS ○ CLUSTER ○ TENSION ○ MIGRAINE ○ NECK ○ TMJ

## Other Symptoms _____

_____

| Triggers | ☁ Weather | Mood before |
|---|---|---|
| ○ Alcohol  ○ Stress at Home | ☐ SUNNY | Headache: |
| ○ Caffeine  ○ Stress at Work | ☐ CLOUDY | ○ Happy |
| ○ Hunger  ○ Eyestrain | ☐ RAINY | ○ Normal |
| ○ Tiredness  ○ Weather | Temp: _____ | ○ Indifferent |
| ○ Allergies  ○ PMS | | ○ Nervous |
| ○ Chocolate  ○ Odor | | ○ Tired |
| ○ Other: _____ | | ○ Sad |

Other: _____

## 💊 Medications & Supplements

_____

_____

_____

_____

_____

### Other Relief Methods:

☐ ICE  ☐ RELAX
☐ HEAT  ☐ OTHER
☐ BED REST
☐ MASSAGE
☐ LOWER LIGHTS

## 🍳 Food Intake _____

_____

_____

_____

_____

_____

## 🌙 Hours of Sleep

_____

## 💧 Water Intake

🍾 🍾 🍾 🍾 🍾

🍾 🍾 🍾 🍾 🍾

# Notes

_____
_____
_____
_____
_____
_____
_____
_____
_____
_____
_____
_____
_____
_____
_____
_____
_____
_____
_____
_____
_____

Date: Start Time: **Severity/Intensity**

End Time: (0) (1) (2) (3) (4) (5)

## Location of headache

○ SINUS  ○ CLUSTER  ○ TENSION  ○ MIGRAINE  ○ NECK  ○ TMJ

## Other Symptoms _____

_____

| Triggers | Weather | Mood before |
|---|---|---|
| | | Headache: |
| ○ Alcohol  ○ Stress at Home | ☐ SUNNY | |
| ○ Caffeine  ○ Stress at Work | ☐ CLOUDY | ○ Happy |
| ○ Hunger  ○ Eyestrain | ☐ RAINY | ○ Normal |
| ○ Tiredness  ○ Weather | Temp: _____ | ○ Indifferent |
| ○ Allergies  ○ PMS | | ○ Nervous |
| ○ Chocolate  ○ Odor | | ○ Tired |
| ○ Other: _____ | | ○ Sad |

Other:

_____

## Medications & Supplements

_____

_____

_____

_____

_____

### Other Relief Methods:

☐ ICE  ☐ RELAX
☐ HEAT  ☐ OTHER
☐ BED REST
☐ MASSAGE
☐ LOWER LIGHTS

## Food Intake _____

_____

_____

_____

_____

_____

## Hours of Sleep

_____

## Water Intake

# Notes

_____

_____

_____

_____

_____

_____

_____

_____

_____

_____

_____

_____

_____

_____

_____

_____

_____

_____

_____

**Date:**      **Start Time:**      **Severity/Intensity**

**End Time:**      (0) (1) (2) (3) (4) (5)

## Location of headache

○ SINUS   ○ CLUSTER   ○ TENSION   ○ MIGRAINE   ○ NECK   ○ TMJ

## Other Symptoms _____

_____

| Triggers | | Weather | Mood before |
|---|---|---|---|
| ○ Alcohol | ○ Stress at Home | ☐ SUNNY | Headache: |
| ○ Caffeine | ○ Stress at Work | ☐ CLOUDY | ○ Happy |
| ○ Hunger | ○ Eyestrain | ☐ RAINY | ○ Normal |
| ○ Tiredness | ○ Weather | Temp: _____ | ○ Indifferent |
| ○ Allergies | ○ PMS | | ○ Nervous |
| ○ Chocolate | ○ Odor | | ○ Tired |
| ○ Other: | | | ○ Sad |

Other:
_____

### Medications & Supplements

_____

_____

_____

_____

_____

### Other Relief Methods:

☐ ICE    ☐ RELAX
☐ HEAT   ☐ OTHER
☐ BED REST
☐ MASSAGE
☐ LOWER LIGHTS

### Food Intake _____

### Hours of Sleep

_____

_____

### Water Intake

_____

_____

_____

# Notes

_____

_____

_____

_____

_____

_____

_____

_____

_____

_____

_____

_____

_____

_____

_____

_____

_____

_____

Date:      Start Time:      Severity/Intensity

End Time:    ⓪ ① ② ③ ④ ⑤

## Location of headache
○ SINUS   ○ CLUSTER   ○ TENSION    ○ MIGRAINE   ○ NECK   ○ TMJ

## Other Symptoms _____

_____

### Triggers
○ Alcohol    ○ Stress at Home
○ Caffeine    ○ Stress at Work
○ Hunger    ○ Eyestrain
○ Tiredness   ○ Weather
○ Allergies   ○ PMS
○ Chocolate   ○ Odor
○ Other: _____

### ☁️Weather
☐ SUNNY
☐ CLOUDY
☐ RAINY
Temp: _____

### Mood before Headache:
○ Happy
○ Normal
○ Indifferent
○ Nervous
○ Tired
○ Sad
Other:

### 💊 Medications & Supplements
_____
_____
_____
_____
_____

### Other Relief Methods:
☐ ICE     ☐ RELAX
☐ HEAT   ☐ OTHER
☐ BED REST
☐ MASSAGE
☐ LOWER LIGHTS

### 🍳 Food Intake _____
_____
_____
_____
_____
_____
_____

### 🌙 Hours of Sleep
_____

### 💧 Water Intake
🍶 🍶 🍶 🍶 🍶

🍶 🍶 🍶 🍶 🍶

# Notes

Date:      Start Time:      Severity/Intensity

End Time:     ⓪ ① ② ③ ④ ⑤

## Location of headache

○ SINUS   ○CLUSTER   ○TENSION   ○MIGRAINE   ○NECK   ○ TMJ

## Other Symptoms _____

_____

| Triggers | | Weather | Mood before |
|---|---|---|---|

### Triggers

○ Alcohol    ○Stress at Home
○Caffeine    ○Stress at Work
○ Hunger    ○Eyestrain
○Tiredness   ○ Weather
○ Allergies   ○ PMS
○ Chocolate ○ Odor
○ Other: _____

### Weather

☐ SUNNY
☐ CLOUDY
☐ RAINY
Temp: _____

### Mood before Headache:

○ Happy
○ Normal
○ Indifferent
○ Nervous
○ Tired
○ Sad
Other: _____

### Medications & Supplements

_____
_____
_____
_____
_____

### Other Relief Methods:

☐ ICE    ☐ RELAX
☐ HEAT   ☐OTHER
☐ BED REST
☐ MASSAGE
☐ LOWER LIGHTS

### Food Intake _____

_____
_____
_____
_____
_____

### Hours of Sleep

_____

### Water Intake

Date:     Start Time:     **Severity/Intensity**

End Time:     (0) (1) (2) (3) (4) (5)

## Location of headache
○ SINUS  ○ CLUSTER  ○ TENSION  ○ MIGRAINE  ○ NECK  ○ TMJ

## Other Symptoms _____

_____

### Triggers
○ Alcohol    ○ Stress at Home
○ Caffeine    ○ Stress at Work
○ Hunger    ○ Eyestrain
○ Tiredness    ○ Weather
○ Allergies    ○ PMS
○ Chocolate    ○ Odor
○ Other: _____

### Weather
☐ SUNNY
☐ CLOUDY
☐ RAINY
Temp: _____

### Mood before Headache:
○ Happy
○ Normal
○ Indifferent
○ Nervous
○ Tired
○ Sad
Other:

## 💊 Medications & Supplements

_____

_____

_____

_____

_____

### Other Relief Methods:
☐ ICE    ☐ RELAX
☐ HEAT    ☐ OTHER
☐ BED REST
☐ MASSAGE
☐ LOWER LIGHTS

## 🍽 Food Intake _____

_____

_____

_____

_____

_____

### 🌙 Hours of Sleep
_____

### 💧 Water Intake
🍶 🍶 🍶 🍶 🍶

🍶 🍶 🍶 🍶 🍶

## Notes

**Date:**      **Start Time:**      **Severity/Intensity**

**End Time:**      ⓪ ① ② ③ ④ ⑤

## Location of headache

○ SINUS ○ CLUSTER ○ TENSION ○ MIGRAINE ○ NECK ○ TMJ

## Other Symptoms _____

_____

### Triggers
○ Alcohol   ○ Stress at Home
○ Caffeine   ○ Stress at Work
○ Hunger   ○ Eyestrain
○ Tiredness   ○ Weather
○ Allergies   ○ PMS
○ Chocolate   ○ Odor
○ Other: _____

### Weather
☐ SUNNY
☐ CLOUDY
☐ RAINY
Temp: _____

### Mood before Headache:
○ Happy
○ Normal
○ Indifferent
○ Nervous
○ Tired
○ Sad
Other: _____

## 💊 Medications & Supplements

_____

_____

_____

_____

_____

### Other Relief Methods:
☐ ICE    ☐ RELAX
☐ HEAT   ☐ OTHER
☐ BED REST
☐ MASSAGE
☐ LOWER LIGHTS

## 🍳 Food Intake _____

_____

_____

_____

_____

_____

### 🌙 Hours of Sleep

_____

### 💧 Water Intake
🍶 🍶 🍶 🍶 🍶

🍶 🍶 🍶 🍶 🍶

# Notes

Date:  Start Time:  Severity/Intensity

End Time:  ⓪ ① ② ③ ④ ⑤

## Location of headache
○ SINUS ○ CLUSTER ○ TENSION ○ MIGRAINE ○ NECK ○ TMJ

## Other Symptoms _____

_____

| ### Triggers | ### ☁ Weather | ### Mood before |
|---|---|---|

### Triggers
○ Alcohol  ○ Stress at Home
○ Caffeine  ○ Stress at Work
○ Hunger  ○ Eyestrain
○ Tiredness  ○ Weather
○ Allergies  ○ PMS
○ Chocolate  ○ Odor
○ Other: _____

### ☁ Weather
☐ SUNNY
☐ CLOUDY
☐ RAINY
Temp: _____

### Mood before Headache:
○ Happy
○ Normal
○ Indifferent
○ Nervous
○ Tired
○ Sad
Other:

### Medications & Supplements

_____
_____
_____
_____
_____

### Other Relief Methods:
☐ ICE     ☐ RELAX
☐ HEAT   ☐ OTHER
☐ BED REST
☐ MASSAGE
☐ LOWER LIGHTS

### Food Intake _____

_____
_____
_____
_____
_____
_____

### ☽ Hours of Sleep

_____

### ○ Water Intake
🍶 🍶 🍶 🍶 🍶

🍶 🍶 🍶 🍶 🍶

Date:     Start Time:     Severity/Intensity

End Time:     (0) (1) (2) (3) (4) (5)

## Location of headache
○ SINUS   ○ CLUSTER   ○ TENSION   ○ MIGRAINE   ○ NECK   ○ TMJ

## Other Symptoms _____

_____

| Triggers | | Weather | Mood before |
|---|---|---|---|
| ○ Alcohol | ○ Stress at Home | ☐ SUNNY | Headache: |
| ○ Caffeine | ○ Stress at Work | ☐ CLOUDY | ○ Happy |
| ○ Hunger | ○ Eyestrain | ☐ RAINY | ○ Normal |
| ○ Tiredness | ○ Weather | Temp: _____ | ○ Indifferent |
| ○ Allergies | ○ PMS | | ○ Nervous |
| ○ Chocolate | ○ Odor | | ○ Tired |
| ○ Other: _____ | | | ○ Sad |

Other: _____

## Medications & Supplements

_____

_____

_____

_____

_____

### Other Relief Methods:
☐ ICE    ☐ RELAX
☐ HEAT   ☐ OTHER
☐ BED REST
☐ MASSAGE
☐ LOWER LIGHTS

## Food Intake _____

_____

_____

_____

_____

_____

_____

## Hours of Sleep

_____

## Water Intake

🍼 🍼 🍼 🍼 🍼

🍼 🍼 🍼 🍼 🍼

## Notes

Date:      Start Time:      Severity/Intensity

End Time:     ⓪ ① ② ③ ④ ⑤

## Location of headache

○ SINUS   ○ CLUSTER   ○ TENSION    ○ MIGRAINE   ○ NECK   ○ TMJ

## Other Symptoms _____

_____

| Triggers | | Weather | Mood before |
|---|---|---|---|
| ○ Alcohol | ○ Stress at Home | ☐ SUNNY | Headache: |
| ○ Caffeine | ○ Stress at Work | ☐ CLOUDY | ○ Happy |
| ○ Hunger | ○ Eyestrain | ☐ RAINY | ○ Normal |
| ○ Tiredness | ○ Weather | Temp: _____ | ○ Indifferent |
| ○ Allergies | ○ PMS | | ○ Nervous |
| ○ Chocolate | ○ Odor | | ○ Tired |
| ○ Other: | | | ○ Sad |

_____    Other:

_____

## 💊 Medications & Supplements

Other Relief
Methods:

_____

_____   ☐ ICE    ☐ RELAX

_____   ☐ HEAT ☐ OTHER

_____   ☐ BED REST

_____   ☐ MASSAGE

_____   ☐ LOWER LIGHTS

## 🍳 Food Intake _____    🌙 Hours of Sleep

_____

_____

_____   💧 Water Intake

_____

_____

_____

_____

# Notes

Date:      Start Time:      Severity/Intensity

End Time:    (0) (1) (2) (3) (4) (5)

## Location of headache

○ SINUS   ○ CLUSTER   ○ TENSION   ○ MIGRAINE   ○ NECK   ○ TMJ

## Other Symptoms _____

_____

### Triggers     ☁Weather     Mood before Headache:

○ Alcohol    ○ Stress at Home    ☐ SUNNY
○ Caffeine    ○ Stress at Work    ☐ CLOUDY    ○ Happy
○ Hunger    ○ Eyestrain    ☐ RAINY    ○ Normal
○ Tiredness    ○ Weather    Temp: _____    ○ Indifferent
○ Allergies    ○ PMS      ○ Nervous
○ Chocolate    ○ Odor      ○ Tired
○ Other: _____      ○ Sad

Other: _____

## 💊 Medications & Supplements

_____
_____
_____
_____
_____

### Other Relief Methods:

☐ ICE    ☐ RELAX
☐ HEAT    ☐ OTHER
☐ BED REST
☐ MASSAGE
☐ LOWER LIGHTS

## 🍽 Food Intake _____

_____
_____
_____
_____
_____

### 🌙 Hours of Sleep

_____

### 💧 Water Intake

🍶 🍶 🍶 🍶 🍶

🍶 🍶 🍶 🍶 🍶

## Notes

Date:      Start Time:      Severity/Intensity

End Time:    ⓪ ① ② ③ ④ ⑤

## Location of headache

○ SINUS   ○ CLUSTER   ○ TENSION   ○ MIGRAINE   ○ NECK   ○ TMJ

## Other Symptoms _____

| Triggers | | ☁☀Weather | Mood before |
|---|---|---|---|
| ○ Alcohol | ○ Stress at Home | ☐ SUNNY | Headache: |
| ○ Caffeine | ○ Stress at Work | ☐ CLOUDY | ○ Happy |
| ○ Hunger | ○ Eyestrain | ☐ RAINY | ○ Normal |
| ○ Tiredness | ○ Weather | Temp: _____ | ○ Indifferent |
| ○ Allergies | ○ PMS | | ○ Nervous |
| ○ Chocolate | ○ Odor | | ○ Tired |
| ○ Other: | | | ○ Sad |

Other: _____

## 💊 Medications & Supplements

_____

_____

_____

_____

_____

### Other Relief Methods:

☐ ICE     ☐ RELAX
☐ HEAT   ☐ OTHER
☐ BED REST
☐ MASSAGE
☐ LOWER LIGHTS

## 🍳 Food Intake _____

_____

_____

_____

_____

_____

## 🌙 Hours of Sleep

_____

## 💧 Water Intake

🍼 🍼 🍼 🍼 🍼

🍼 🍼 🍼 🍼 🍼

**Date:**     **Start Time:**     **Severity/Intensity**

**End Time:**     (0) (1) (2) (3) (4) (5)

## Location of headache
○ SINUS   ○ CLUSTER   ○ TENSION    ○ MIGRAINE   ○ NECK   ○ TMJ

## Other Symptoms _____

_____

| Triggers | Weather | Mood before Headache: |
|---|---|---|
| ○ Alcohol   ○ Stress at Home | ☐ SUNNY | ○ Happy |
| ○ Caffeine   ○ Stress at Work | ☐ CLOUDY | ○ Normal |
| ○ Hunger   ○ Eyestrain | ☐ RAINY | ○ Indifferent |
| ○ Tiredness   ○ Weather | Temp: _____ | ○ Nervous |
| ○ Allergies   ○ PMS | | ○ Tired |
| ○ Chocolate   ○ Odor | | ○ Sad |
| ○ Other: _____ | | Other: _____ |

## Medications & Supplements

_____

_____

_____

_____

_____

### Other Relief Methods:
☐ ICE    ☐ RELAX
☐ HEAT   ☐ OTHER
☐ BED REST
☐ MASSAGE
☐ LOWER LIGHTS

## Food Intake _____

_____

_____

_____

_____

_____

## Hours of Sleep

_____

## Water Intake

🍶 🍶 🍶 🍶 🍶

🍶 🍶 🍶 🍶 🍶

# Notes

Date: Start Time: **Severity/Intensity**

End Time: (0) (1) (2) (3) (4) (5)

## Location of headache

○ SINUS ○ CLUSTER ○ TENSION ○ MIGRAINE ○ NECK ○ TMJ

## Other Symptoms _____

_____

| Triggers | Weather | Mood before Headache: |
|---|---|---|
| ○ Alcohol ○ Stress at Home | ☐ SUNNY | ○ Happy |
| ○ Caffeine ○ Stress at Work | ☐ CLOUDY | ○ Normal |
| ○ Hunger ○ Eyestrain | ☐ RAINY | ○ Indifferent |
| ○ Tiredness ○ Weather | Temp: _____ | ○ Nervous |
| ○ Allergies ○ PMS | | ○ Tired |
| ○ Chocolate ○ Odor | | ○ Sad |
| ○ Other: _____ | | Other: |

## Medications & Supplements

_____

_____

_____

_____

_____

### Other Relief Methods:

☐ ICE ☐ RELAX
☐ HEAT ☐ OTHER
☐ BED REST
☐ MASSAGE
☐ LOWER LIGHTS

## Food Intake _____

## Hours of Sleep

_____

_____

### Water Intake

_____

_____

_____

_____

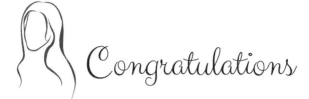

# Congratulations

YOU HAVE SUCCESSFULLY
COMPLETED YOUR JOURNAL!!! IF YOU
LOVED YOUR JOURNAL PLEASE COME
BACK TO OUR STORE!

SCAN QR CODE

Printed in Great Britain
by Amazon

25740995R00066